The Healing Codes
Underlying Principles

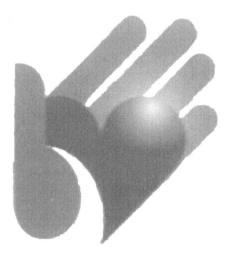

by Dr. Jerry Graham
www.healingcodes777.com

ISBN: 1463692935

ISBN-13: 978-1463692933

Dedication

This book is dedicated to my incredible wife, Sharon, for her infinite patience and amazing good will.

Contents

Preface

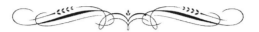

Early in 2003, I received an unsolicited invitation to be part of a pioneering group of coaches working with a newly discovered technique in the energy healing arena. Prior to that invitation, I had never even heard of energy healing, energy medicine, energy psychology, or any of the other variations of the application of energy to deal with the body's physical and mental issues.

As a university-trained engineer who had recently begun a second career in the ministry with an emphasis in Life Coaching, I was the original skeptic. This notion of using the energy present within each of us stretched any of my training way beyond credibility. While I wasn't one of those who was fearful of New Age thinking, I was quite concerned about the foundation of this strange, new (to me) technology.

After an incredible amount of soul searching, I decided to "stick my toe into the water" and attend the initial training session in Nashville, TN. While there I had the opportunity to meet Dr. Alex Loyd and others who had been practicing this particular energy technique for the previous year and found them to all be extremely credible and excited about the results they had seen both in themselves and in those they had worked with.

I took the plunge and began the training to become one of the charter members of the certified Healing Codes coaches and began working with clients. In the years since, I have worked with over three hundred clients, many of whom have seen incredible results due to their use of the codes. It has been incredibly gratifying to say the least. However, as with anything that requires a certain amount of faith and discipline to get started, there have been some who have not seen results they had hoped for, most often I would surmise because they weren't faithful in their use of the codes and/or they gave up "just inches away from the gold." Very sad indeed.

The following chapters are compiled from the notes I took through a series of lectures given by Dr. Loyd regarding some of the underlying principles behind The Healing Codes. I found the lectures to be extremely helpful in my understanding of the mechanism of the codes and sincerely hope that my notes on those lectures will be of use to you as well.

If you're already using The Healing Codes, I pray that this information will increase your commitment to be even more consistent with your use of the codes. If you're not yet a user, I sincerely hope that what follows will open your mind to give them a try. The Healing Codes as an organization has one of the most liberal guarantees I have ever seen, allowing you one full year to try the codes with absolutely no risk on your part. You've got everything to gain and nothing to lose.

To experience The Healing Codes for yourself, go to www.HealingCodes777.com.

God bless you,
Dr. Jerry Graham, Ph.D., D.Min.

1 The Unacceptably High Cost of Living in Fear

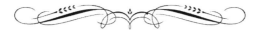

Fear and Anxiety Are Everywhere

Have you noticed that fear seems to be settling in for a long visit? A quick glance at the news tells us that many people are fearful about the economy, their investments, and whether their jobs will survive this downturn. We hear stories every day about people losing their homes or jobs. Widespread financial disaster appears to be looming on the horizon.

And that's just the economy! So many other issues – terrorism, hunger and crime, to name a few, have more people than ever living in a state of unease.

The Cost: Stress and Disease

And there's a cost to all that fear – anxiety, depression, and stress are escalating in response to external factors that seem to be out of our control.

What's the result of that escalation? It's an astronomical increase in the incidence of disease. Equally troubling is the accompanying increase in the amount being spent for health care.

Here's some alarming information to illustrate what all this fear is doing to our bodies:

- In 1971, cancer was the eighth leading cause of death in the United States. It's now number two and recently predicted to become the world's top killer by 2010!
- The skyrocketing amount of money being spent on mental and physical health is now over-stressing the Medicaid and Medicare systems. According to ABC News, thirty billion dollars are being spent every year for prescription drugs alone. That's a 330% increase since 1977!

The End Result: Crisis in Healthcare Industry

What's the end result of this fear/illness cycle? One thing is clear; we now face a healthcare system in absolute chaos. Consider the reports being issued almost weekly refuting the benefits of drugs once thought to be therapeutic. We're now finding that original medication studies were skewed by withheld data! With our own bodies succumbing to the effects of fear and stress, and our healthcare system crumbling around us, what can be done to bring us back to health?

Possible Solution Number 1

There are two solutions available right now to anyone willing to take advantage of them. The first is what Dr. Alex, founder of The Healing Codes, calls "living from the heart." In a nutshell, this means being willing to face the chaos in our lives, in truth and in love. Dr. Bruce Lipton, author of *The Biology of Belief,* has found in his research over the years that ninety-five percent of disease comes, not from genetics, but from our own internal programming.

Consider the implications of Dr. Lipton's findings – the diseases which seem to be overtaking us are not, for the most part, coming from external circumstances, but rather from what's going on inside us. It's not a question of will I get cancer, or will I get diabetes, or will I get whatever – you already have those diseases in your body. The question is more one of will stress "unmask" or break down the body's natural immune response so that those diseases begin to manifest?

In order to bring healing to our souls and bodies, we must be willing to change the programming, or response, to the chaos around us. Will those external factors change? Maybe not, but when we begin to approach the stresses of life from a place of peace, love, and health, we begin to heal our own bodies.

Possible Solution Number 2

Another remedy to the stress that kills us is the "energy medicine" which God built into nature to allow us to heal ourselves. At the mere mention of energy medicine, many people recoil in fear that this is one of those spooky approaches that has no basis in science. Just for the record, Dr. Mehmet Oz, author of the "New York Time's" best seller *You: The Owner's Manual*, and an almost weekly guest on the Oprah show, wrote in his book that the next big frontier in medicine is energy medicine. Why would a prominent, traditional medical practitioner like Dr. Oz subject himself to the probable ridicule of his colleagues unless he accepted the fact that what Albert Einstein told us about energy was true? It seems that almost every other scientific field except medicine has begun to make drastic changes in recognition that everything is energy. It's also significant to understand that the most sophisticated diagnostic equipment used by the medical profession on a daily basis is in fact based on energy principles. CT Scanners, MRI devices, et.al., are all simply measuring energy.

Based upon quantum physics, energy medicine works at the cellular level to bring about change. Imagine breaking our dependence on our ailing health care medicine and instead, choosing to use this God-given tool for healing. Energy medicine is no replacement for living from the heart, but it is another tool we can use to move ourselves toward healing.

What is the cost of living in constant fear? Depression, despair, and illness. But there's hope! The fear we're living in now doesn't have to control future health and happiness. We already have the tools available to face the storms that come into our lives. By learning to live from the heart, and taking advantage of the power of energy medicine, we can break the grip of fear and begin to heal its effect on our bodies.

2 Unconscious Intention Trumps Conscious Intentions

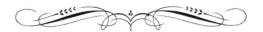

If you're like many of us, at some point you've visited a bookstore hoping to find the answer to a problem in your life. Self-help books and recordings abound and, predictably, they define the source of our problems several different ways.

Let's narrow down our focus to the five main causes for our problems that most self-help writers cite. Those are: physiology, behaviors, thinking patterns, emotions, and conscious beliefs. What you'll find offered by most writers as a root cause to life's difficulties falls into those five categories.

A second opinion

Another school of thought says that while it's true you may be able to change yourself to some extent by addressing deficiencies in those areas, those inadequacies are actually symptoms of a much deeper problem.

What that means is that lasting change cannot be

accomplished in life until you recognize the true source of your problems, rather than simply identifying the symptoms. Unless we're able to go directly to the root of problem areas in our lives, we continue to deal with symptoms which tend to return.

Think of it as a tree with a deep taproot. If the tree becomes diseased, you can choose to cut it off at the ground (get rid of the obvious symptom), but new shoots will probably appear from what's unseen under the ground. You can, however, dig out the taproot as well as cutting down the tree and completely remove the disease.

Lasting change – the true goal

Here's another way to think of it: we've heard a great deal recently about "conscious intention" and its power to bring about change. Unfortunately, conscious intention or "willpower" doesn't always bring about *lasting* change. If it did, we'd all be skinny, happy, and rich!

The reason conscious intentions alone don't bring permanent change is that they seek to overcome symptoms, not cure the root source. When that fails to make us happy, we usually move on to any number of negative behaviors that move us further away from peace and satisfaction.

When all else fails...blame!

One of the things we tend to do when our conscious intentions don't overcome damaging behavior is to turn the spotlight on someone else's behavior. Blaming someone else for our life's failures is much easier than looking for the root causes of them. Becoming judgmental, however, actually just adds another layer of pain in our relationships instead of solving our problems. Whether we blame a politician, a spouse, or even God for our pain, it's still a negative behavior that moves us farther away from solutions.

Intentions – Conscious or Unconscious?

Doesn't it make sense to instead find and deal with the root causes? To begin to do that, we must first identify the things that are blocking us from life and health. Those stumbling blocks are our "unconscious intentions." If those unconscious intentions don't match the efforts of our willpower, we're doomed to failure!

As Dr. Alex reports, scientific research has already proven that basing your future happiness on conscious intention almost never brings the results you desire. The key to lasting happiness in life is in aligning what we really want (our unconscious intentions) with what we say we want (our conscious intentions). Only then can all our energy be focused on improving our lives.

Dr. Alex tells of the opportunity he had to spend the better part of a day with Dr. William Tiller, professor emeritus of Materials Science and Engineering at Stanford University and one of the featured experts in the film "What the Bleep Do We Know?". Dr. Tiller verified the importance and power of conscious intention, but went on to point out that we all also have an unconscious intention, and that if the two do not agree, the unconscious intention will win *every* time.

Dr. Bruce Lipton has in essence said that it is almost impossible to change things by willpower. As important and necessary as willpower is, unconscious intention is one million times more powerful than willpower or conscious intention. That's why so few people ever "break the cycle" of changing the negative patterns that run in their lives. Many experts conclude that people just don't ever change.

As a blanket statement, it can be said that every

program that attributes problems to something that you must change by will power simply doesn't work to bring about long-term change. We can't throw away willpower and conscious intention, but it's vital that we take steps to fix the unconscious intention so as to bring it into alignment with the conscious intention.

Once we're willing to stop blaming others and stop focusing on the symptoms instead of the source of our problems, we've taken the first step to finding health, peace, and happiness in our lives. Commit to discovering the deeply embedded roots that anchor you to unhappiness, and begin focusing your energy on healing that pain for good.

3 Stress and Failure Come From a Physical Source

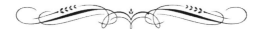

Symptoms are a diversion

What will it take to break the cycle of failure in your life? Many of us spend years, and substantial amounts of money, attempting to cure one of the five major areas in which problems occur.

Whether we focus on our beliefs, behaviors, physical ailments, emotional problems, or negative thoughts, though, we're really just dealing with symptoms, rather than identifying the root cause. Sometimes that struggle to change symptomatic behavior becomes a substitute for finding, and dealing with, the real reason we continue to fail.

Stress is the real culprit

It should encourage you to know that research now shows us that there is an actual physical cause for this cycle of struggle and defeat. We now know, that the bottom line cause for failure in our lives is *stress*. In fact, the Centers for Disease Control in Atlanta, reported that ninety percent of disease, is brought about by stress.

As we saw in the first chapter, Dr. Bruce Lipton, a groundbreaking cell biologist, goes farther and concludes that ninety-five percent of disease is caused by stress, and that the other five percent that is 'genetic' is the result of an ancestor experiencing enough stress to unmask a disease at the cellular level and introduce it into the family's genetics.

Stop and think about that for a minute. What if we could literally break the cycle of genetically inherited disease by addressing the response to stress in the current generation? Think of the impact that would have on our future.

Stress – How it works

Let's explore then, how stress actually brings about disease and failure in our lives. It's important to know that stress actually does five things – it makes us physically ill, drains our energy, gives us over to a negative outlook, reduces our problem solving ability, and because of these other results, predicts our failure.

What is the most common response to this impact? We try to "will" our way back into health. Recall the discussion in the previous chapter about conscious intention and willpower. Imagine being asked to constantly push a heavy object up an incline. That's what it's like when we confront the effects of stress with our own willpower. We chase the latest self-help book, we pray, we take more and more medication to relieve our symptoms. Failure however, is inevitable until we find the root cause of all that stress!

I know what to do, but I don't know why I don't do it

Dr. Alex learned in his private counseling practice that 99% of the time, his patients could answer accurately when asked what they should do differently. They couldn't however, answer the question, "Why, then, aren't you doing what you need to be doing?" They either didn't know why, or they didn't believe they were capable of doing what needed to be done.

Here's the lesson: it is almost impossible to heal deeply held deficiencies by our own willpower. So, how is it possible to be released from the cycle of sickness and failure?

What was meant to save us is now killing us

For the answer, we have to look to our own brains. When we experience stress, the hypothalamus signals the pituitary to redirect blood flow from our internal organs toward the large muscle groups. This is the original "fight or flight" response that kept our ancestors alive. The only time that response was supposed to go into action was when we felt the imminent danger of physical death. In modern life, however, this response is triggered when we experience a *perceived* threat. Think of how your body responds to a verbal confrontation. Muscles tense, breathing gets shallow, body is ready for action.

That physical reaction is caused by the cortisol that's being sent through the body by the pituitary. What's even more important is what happens to the cells that are being deprived of blood and oxygen. They are moving toward critical cellular stress. We are actually experiencing a momentary malfunction of the immune system. The cellular stress brought about by this reaction, "unmasks" the possibility of disease in individual cells. We literally "open the door" to the diseases that lie dormant in our body by reacting to stress over and over throughout the day.

Therefore, since we know that the actual physical cause of our relational, physical, and emotional problems is stress, we can also know how to heal ourselves. We must begin by identifying the root cause of our stress and learn how to lessen its impact on our lives.

For your further growth

What is it in your day that causes you to feel your stress level rising? Is it the bills? Thinking about your bank account? Going to your job? Dealing with an obstinate family member or work colleague? The fact that your spouse doesn't put the cap back on the toothpaste? Most people can identify 20 or 30 things that literally cause them to feel their stress level increasing. We suggest you take the time to make a list

If your stress level is indeed going up from the items on this list, according to the definition of the fight or flight response, somewhere deep inside you, you are believing that each of these items is going to literally cause you to physically die within the next few minutes. In other words, you are unconsciously believing the lie that those items on your list are going to kill you. Since this is a ridiculous conclusion when framed in that way, does it not become abundantly clear that you are dealing with some internal programming that is causing you to go into stress?

4 How to Activate the Success Mechanism

If it were suddenly announced that a pill had been developed that would make us successful, the road to the nearest pharmacy would be clogged with traffic! Many of us struggle to find success in our lives, but haven't found a way to make it ours. What if I told you that the key to lifelong success already exists, and it resides within our own bodies?

The Failure Response

To illustrate how that's possible, we need to first look at what causes us to fail. Research has proven that the "failure mechanism" is kicked into gear when we face stress in our lives. The chain of events is like this – we face a perceived threat (someone else's anger, a high pressure work situation, etc.), and as described in the last chapter, our body responds to it in the same way that our ancestor's bodies responded to a physical threat of death. The hypothalamus in the brain tells our pituitary gland to rally the adrenal system to release cortisol and adrenaline throughout our bodies, making us ready to fight, or run from the fight.

The result of that constant stress reaction literally

weakens our immune systems, dulls our intelligence, heightens our awareness of pain, drains our energy, raises our blood pressure, destroys our ability to relate to other people, brings about negative behaviors like deceit, fear, and suspicion, and, if that's not enough, closes off nutrition to our very cells and makes them the perfect environment for the growth of disease! Is it any wonder we struggle to be healthy, happy, and successful?

A Better Alternative

What if, instead of our bodies being in a constant state of anxious high alert from all that cortisol pumping through us, we could find a way to use the hypothalamus/pituitary/adrenal gland cycle to bring about success? That's possible, because our bodies already contain the hormone oxytocin, which allows us to respond favorably to stressful situations. All we need is a way to release oxytocin, rather than cortisol, into our bodies in response to daily stress.

Before you learn to trigger the success response, start by answering a question. What do you truly want out of life? Dr. Alex learned through interviews with hundreds of people that what most people want is health, success, or good relationships with other people.

Success Response Benefits

The fact is that our physiological response to stress has a major impact in each of those areas. If, as we learned, our body's "failure response" negatively impacts those things immediately, it stands to reason that a physical "success response" should have an immediate positive impact as well. Swedish medical doctor and physiologist Kerstin Uvnas Moberg, and author of *The Oxytocin Factor: Tapping the Hormone of Calm, Love, and Healing,* as well as several other prominent researchers and practitioners, report that people who learn to trigger oxytocin rather than adrenaline when stressed experience many of the following benefits:

- Enhanced relationships
- Feelings of love, joy, and peace
- Increased immune function
- Reduced stress
- Lowered blood pressure
- Counteraction to the addiction/withdrawal cycle
- Stimulated human growth hormone to reverse aging
- Increased trust & wise judgment
- Modulated appetite and digestion

- Promotes healing
- Stimulates relaxation and non-stress energy to allow energy/sleep balance
- Stimulates higher neurological activity such as problem solving
- Opens our cells to nutrition and health

If you knew how to bring about these benefits, instead of constantly experiencing failure, wouldn't you choose to live in success? Dr. Alex tells us that it's possible for every one of us.

You Already Know How

You're probably already activating the success response temporarily through pleasurable experiences such as sex and eating. That's why we love to do those things! We get a momentary glimpse of what it is to feel great.

But there's a healthy way to make that feeling a regular part of our lives. According to a study conducted by Dr. Rebecca Turner and her colleagues (www.oxytocin.org/oxytoc/), to turn on the success response, we must simply learn how to recall a pleasant relationship experience that is not overshadowed by negative relationship experiences. Activating that memory of a positive, loving relationship stimulates the release of oxytocin to our bodies.

If loving relationship memories are stifled by negative ones, those negative memories must first be healed. Dr. Alex teaches The Healing Codes participants to heal those negative memories, and then infuse "true love memories" to bring about that positive, healthy success response. When our hearts are cleared of the negative garbage and we begin to activate happy, loving memories, we can live permanently in success and health.

For your further growth

You may think that sitting around reminiscing about pleasant experiences is a total waste of time, but I propose that if you proactively clear out the negative memories first and then recall those positive memories of love, joy, and peace, that you will begin to notice a difference in your overall life, not just while thinking about the good memories. What few people understand is that memories, good or bad, are broadcasting like little TV stations throughout the body 24 hours a day, 7 days a week.

We invite you to make a list of the five memories that are most painful to you. Then recognize that based on our TV station analogy, that those memories are actively causing internal stress even when you aren't actively thinking about them. Is it any wonder that you seem to be in a constant state of stress?

The good news is that there are ways that you can proactively go about healing, or erasing the negative effects, of those radiators of distress. Once you have "turned down the volume" on the negative, you make room for the positive memories to radiate positivity on a 24/7 basis. Since this is going on even when you are not thinking about it, you can clearly see that this goes far beyond the power of positive thinking.

5 Beliefs – The Reason We Do What We Do

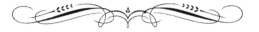

Why do we continue to do things that are self-destructive? Whether in relationships, health, or finances, many of us remain trapped in patterns of negative behavior that bring the worst possible results. What have scientists learned that might help us break these destructive patterns, once and for all?

The Healing Power of Beliefs

One area under much scrutiny in traditional and alternative medical circles is the power of a person's internal beliefs to impact their physiology. You may already be familiar with the placebo effect, but here's some new information that may startle you. In January of 2008, major news outlets began to report about a groundbreaking clinical study on the use of placebos. (http://www.time.com/time/health/article/0,8599,1700079,00.html, http://www.bloomberg.com/apps/news?pid=20601203&sid=andNe8m1qt_k&refer=insurance, et al.) Almost fifty percent of the doctors in the survey reported prescribing placebos over the previous year. When asked why they would prescribe a placebo to a patient, ninety-six percent of the doctors doing so said they believed they would see a clinical, therapeutic result after prescribing a placebo. In other words, because their *patients believed* they would feel relief after taking a sugar pill, their bodies actually felt relief. Their patients' bodies actually produced a healing effect based upon their belief that the placebo would work.

Beliefs Become Physical

What does that research tell us about the mind's ability to impact a person's daily actions? If we can feel physical relief from symptoms because we believe we will, doesn't it make sense that our physical actions are also a result of what we believe? Here's how Dr. Alex expresses it, "Everything a person does, they do because they believe they should."

Before you dismiss his statement, recall that back in chapter 3 we briefly referred to Dr. Alex's private counseling practice where he observed that 99% of the time, his patients could answer accurately when asked what they should do differently. But they couldn't answer the next logical question, "Why, then, aren't you doing what you need to be doing?" They either didn't know why, or they didn't believe they were capable of doing what needed to be done.

Recall also that we have conscious beliefs as well as un- and subconscious beliefs. When we are challenged to look at our beliefs, we are only capable, by definition, of looking at those that are in our conscious mind. The alarming fact is that 99% of our beliefs are in our un- and subconscious mind making them impossible to examine, even though according to Dr. Bruce Lipton they are a million times more powerful in regulating our behavior that our conscious beliefs.

Think of some common examples from your own experience. Have you ever known that you should exercise regularly but yet not been able to consistently exercise? All kind of reasons (excuses?) come up to take us off the hook. Isn't the same true of our eating habits? We know that the apple is better for us than the donut, but what do most of us end up reaching for? Is it possible that deep down we have a belief that says we shouldn't have to exercise or that somewhere deep in our subconscious there is a belief that eating that donut will serve us more than eating the apple?

When we have conflicting beliefs about something,

the strongest underlying belief is what drives our actions in that area. This should open your mind to the reality that it's not always conscious thoughts that control us! Our most deeply-held beliefs may be hidden within the unconscious mind, sabotaging healthy behaviors and frustrating our efforts to "will" our way past negative ones.

Change the Belief to Change the Action

Dr. Lipton found in his research that a person's beliefs control their physical response to everyday stress, which in turn, determines their overall health. By changing our most basic beliefs, he determined, we can change our physical response to life. What we can conclude from his research and all the other studies mentioned is that, if we can control our health with our beliefs, we can also stop negative behaviors by changing those same beliefs. That, in fact, is the only way to bring about lasting change. Until we learn to recognize and heal our unconscious negative beliefs, we will never live healthy, successful lives. The lesson to take with you is this – if you continually do things that are destructive to your personal peace, that's an indicator that your underlying belief system is in need of healing. Once you accept the truth of that, you can start taking the steps to move toward health, happiness, and peace of mind.

For Your Further Growth

In light of the above, how can you determine what you really believe? The answer is to simply observe what you feel and what you do, regardless of what you consciously believe.

Ask yourself, am I doing in my life, 100%, the things I want to be doing? Am I exercising as much as I believe I should be? Am I eating as well nutritionally as I think I should be eating? Are you devoting as much time to work and to spiritual pursuits as you believe you should be? Are you doing the things for your spouse that you know that if you do would light up his/her eyes? Are you spending as much time with your children as you know you should be spending? Are you as successful as you believe you should be? Do you see a way that if you did things differently you would probably be more successful?

So now the next question to ask your self is, why? You just said that you believe it, so why aren't you doing it? Most will answer, I don't know or I can't. When you have something in your life where you're not doing what you believe you should be (or vice-versa), it is a virtual certainty that you have a belief in your un- or subconscious mind that says, don't do that.

Now the question becomes, why in the world would you have a belief that tells you not to do something that when you examine it rationally would be a good thing to do? The surprising and somewhat disconcerting fact of the matter is that the un- and subconscious mind are irrational a lot of the time.

Your un- and subconscious mind is designed to protect you. That is why you can be convinced that a stick is a snake and react as if it were a snake. You can be convinced that a thunderstorm is imminent danger. That's why those suffering from anorexia can look in a mirror and be absolutely convinced that they are grossly overweight.

You can absolutely rest assured that for everything you are doing (or not doing), that you have a belief in your un- or subconscious that says, do that. There are a thousand reasons, e.g., it's dangerous for some reason, it won't make any difference, It won't make any difference if I put in all those hours at work to succeed because I'm just the kind of person that will not succeed no matter what I do. My appearance works against me, I'm not talented enough, I'm not connected enough, I never could measure up to my sibling or in school, so I'm obviously never going to measure up in anything.

All this is to say that for us to do what we know we need to do and not do the opposite, there is no possible solution that does not involve healing the beliefs in the un- and subconscious mind because they are dictating the feelings and behavior and thoughts that are acted on by the conscious mind and that ultimately change the very physiology of the body.

So, we invite you to make a list of those areas in your life where you are not doing what you know you should be doing in your rational mind, and secondly, write down how your life would be different if you were doing those things that you know you should be doing.

6 How to Build the Success Foundation

Core Beliefs by Six

Here's something to think about: every human being has a stimulus response programming system that is the basis for his reactions to what goes on around him. During the first six years of life, we form core beliefs about danger and safety. We do, of course, add layers of new information to those beliefs as we mature, but what if the foundation itself is flawed?

If you've ever been in an area during a landslide, you might see houses clinging to the side of a hill, barely supported by their foundations. That's what a shaky core belief system looks like in a person's life. For example: you walk into a social situation and feel terrified, although no one there is behaving threateningly. You've just reacted to a faulty stimulus response system. Your response to the circumstance is based on false beliefs.

Stress Results from Faulty Core Beliefs

That false programming, deep in our hearts, impacts our rational belief system to the point many of us can feel physically threatened by a harmless audience. Those lies about what is real are constantly reactivated by new situations. Most of us, though, can't articulate that, so we rationalize by saying we don't have a certain talent, or that we aren't feeling well. The truth is that we don't feel well because a lie in our hearts is making us behave irrationally!

Why is this foundation so powerful? According to Dr. Alex Loyd, who has spent years reviewing scientific research while formulating The Healing Codes, if the brain senses fear, it initiates the stress response throughout the body. If the brain senses love without fear, it initiates the "Success Response." He believes that physiological success response, including the release of oxytocin into the body, opens the door to success, happiness, health, and better relationships.

Fear Not!

If he's correct, the solution, then, is to have strong foundational beliefs that are not based upon fear. It's no coincidence that in the Bible we find the phrase "fear not" 365 times! The Biblical response to life's stresses, whether financial, relational, or any other perceived threat, is that fear isn't necessary. In combination with the current scientific data on the impact of fear on our bodies, we begin to understand the benefit in pursuing that mindset!

If fear can be defined as a programmed reaction to real or perceived pain, then anger is what occurs when the thing we feared actually happens. If we're spending our days imagining bad things happening, and becoming angry about it, there's a faulty image in our hearts about what is real.

Down the Rabbit Hole We Go

Let's go a little further. Sadness occurs when the action of our anger doesn't change our negative circumstances. We move into shame when we decide it's our fault that fear, anger, and sadness have come into our lives. What a painful, negative cycle – and it all starts with a false belief about our circumstances.

How to know if you're caught in this cycle? If you live in a state of unease, rather than peace, your life is probably based on a faulty set of foundational beliefs. So, what's the cure? First, we learn to tell ourselves the truth about the circumstances we're in. We say things like, "When I step up to the podium, no one is going to physically attack me."

Before we can speak rational truth into our emotions,

though, we must cure the deep, hidden lies that live in our hearts. Once we recognize, and begin to heal those faulty beliefs, we are free to build a foundation of love and truth. When that happens, the physical stress response that often brings about failure is interrupted and we begin to experience true success.

7 Stress Reaction – The Physical Source of Disease

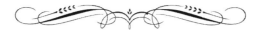

Stress from Wrong Beliefs

For decades, scientists have understood the "stress reaction" that triggers a powerful physical response throughout our bodies. As we discussed in chapter 3 we already know from this research that the constant triggering of the stress reaction day after day can have a negative impact on our health.

But what actually causes that stress reaction to trigger in the first place? Dr. Alex tells us that the cause is a set of faulty beliefs that bring about excessive fear and anger. Here's another way to look at it – King Solomon told us three thousand years ago to "guard the heart above all else, for from it flows everything else in life."

What that means is that "the heart," where our most deeply-held beliefs are stored, must be accurate because from those beliefs comes either a healthy life or the problems that plague us. In other words, it's the wrong beliefs we hold within ourselves that are the very core of the excessive stress that brings destruction into our lives.

Fear, Anger, Stress and Cellular Memories

But what does science have to say about the root cause of fear, stress, and disease? Dr. Eric Nessler of the University of Texas Southwest Medical Center in Dallas is quoted as saying on the Dallas Morning News in 2004, "For many diseases, treatments today aren't much better than Band-Aids. They address the disease's symptoms, but not its cause. Harnessing this knowledge offers the potential of really correcting the abnormality."

The abnormality he's referring to is genetically-based disease! He goes on to say that healing diseases such as cancer may be the result of replacing negative cellular memories with positive ones and that "...scientists are striving to understand how cells acquire these memories and perhaps treat disease at its root by adjusting them."

Dr. Nessler isn't the only scientist making these claims. John Sarno, MD at NYU's Langone Medical Center, tells us that adult chronic pain and illness is caused by fear and anger in the unconscious mind. He defines that fear and anger as "cellular memories" and further says that those memories must be healed to end the pain and disease.

Healing Cellular Memories Is the Key

To tie all this together, Dr. Lipton explains that ninety-five percent of disease is related to stress and fear, and the rest is caused by the unmasking of a disease gene by stress somewhere in our ancestry. Because our very cells hold the residue of fear and anger, healing involves removing the beliefs that trigger stress. As we learn from Dr. Lipton's research, that process requires much more than willpower. It requires a structured "reprogramming" of our most basic beliefs about ourselves.

These studies offer all of us tremendous hope. They give scientific proof that taking the steps to learn to "live from the heart" and heal the deeply-rooted false beliefs keeping us in a constant state of fear and stress is the key to living a genuinely healthy life.

For Your Further Growth

Stress immediately suppresses our immune system. Then it "dumbs" us down, drains our energy, and causes us to view things from a negative perspective. This occurs as the hypothalamus senses a threat or any emotion that has its root in fear (e.g., anger, sadness, low self-worth, overwhelm, frustration, and many, many others).

Most think that the "stress switch" is thrown by the hypothalamus only when one consciously is thinking about or remembering the negative memory. Unfortunately, that's not at all true. These negative memories are like little radio or TV stations transmitting those emotions 24/7 to the cells around them, shifting the cells from growth mode to self-protect mode.

These signals are also picked up by the hypothalamus which dutifully flips that "stress switch." So it should be obvious that the thing that must change to eliminate the stress is not the hypothalamus (which is there for a life-saving purpose), but the negative memories which are broadcasting the stress producing signals.

This demonstrates that you can force positive thoughts and do positive affirmations all day long with negligible long-term effect, because the root of the stress is occurring in the un- and subconscious and are orders of magnitude stronger than the conscious mind can counteract. In actual fact, the negative memories are protected from being altered because they are providing the body the first line of defense from whatever created the memory from happening again.

8 Healing the Images in Our Hearts

Research is showing more clearly all the time that an unhealthy body is the result of faulty beliefs which bring about constant stress. But have you ever stopped to think how those beliefs are stored within your body in the first place?

Images Stored in Our Cells

A number of respected clinical studies have shown that our most deeply held beliefs are stored as cellular memory, rather than conscious thought. To fully understand this concept you should know that these beliefs, these cellular memories, are stored as images.

Pierce Howard, in *The Owner's Manual for the Brain*, expands on this concept by saying that data is also recalled by our brains as a series of images. In other words, the images our experiences create are held in storage within our cells, to be recalled when we need them to understand the world.

Cellular Memories as Thoughts

Antonio Damasio, Director of the Brain and Creativity Institute at the University of Southern California, explains it this way, "The ability to display images internally and order those images in a process is called thought." In other words, the thought processes of the mind work in association with the images we store at the cellular level.

Those images, by the way, are a universal language. When we don't speak the language of another country, we usually resort to symbols to get our point across. This reinforces the fact that all people, no matter what language they speak, store data from their life experiences as a collection of images.

"Imageless thought" is, in fact, impossible. Your eyes pick up an image and send it on to your cells to store. When you're in a situation that makes you recall that image, your mind compares the stored image against the current situation. This happens so that your body is constantly prepared to defend itself, run away from the situation, or stay neutral.

Because that's true, your beliefs about your past experiences must also be stored in those images. So doesn't it make sense that if you stored a negative image about something that's actually harmless, your mind would always jump to the wrong conclusion? Those wrong conclusions lead to the constant stress that keeps many people unhealthy.

Unhealthy Images, Unhealthy Response

Let's use an example provided by Dr. Alex Loyd, founder of The Healing Codes; if, as a child, you see Santa Claus for the first time, your mind creates an image of the concept "Santa Claus" and stores it. Every time you hear the words "Santa Claus" thereafter, your mind pulls up that image you've stored.

If that image is a positive one, hearing the words "Santa Claus" will cause the brain to trigger a pleasurable response. If it's a negative cellular memory, those same words will trigger the stress response, instead. Until you intentionally change that image, you'll be trapped with a negative response to a harmless situation.

Heal the Image, Heal the Body

Given that scientifically proven information, we now know the only permanent way to heal our bodies is to heal these negative cellular memories. It's what Dr. Loyd refers to as "living from the heart", rather than being trapped in automatic negative responses. Once we do, we'll have positive, appropriate images available for our minds to use. As a result, we experience peace, health, and happiness instead of illness and defeat.

Doesn't that sound much better than treating the symptoms which plague us? Embracing this simple fact can be life-changing. If we heal the heart, that immense storehouse of images from our lives, our bodies will be healed, at last.

9 The Power of Living From the Heart

If you're constantly experiencing stress, and you're also struggling with destructive habits, you should know there's a connection between the two. While we might think that our stress is caused by our bad habits, though, the exact opposite is actually true.

Faulty Memories Equal Faulty Responses

We've learned from recent scientific research that our brains respond to our environment based on images stored at the cellular level. When those images, those cellular memories, are faulty, we respond negatively to people, things, or situations that won't physically harm us. That's called "stress."

Millions of dollars have been spent seeking ways to "de-stress" ourselves and correct negative habits, but little permanent change is seen in most people's lives.

Why Conscious Intention Won't Work

You've probably heard a lot in the past few years about the power of "conscious intention." The movie "The

Secret" details the ways in which conscious intention can be used to significantly change a person's life.

Here's the problem-our conscious minds don't control our external behavior! That may be hard to take, since we'd like to believe that we consciously control what we choose to do each day. But that simply isn't true.

Research has proven that at least ninety-five percent of the time, most of us are operating within our unconscious or subconscious minds. Simply put, that means the majority of our behavior is driven by what lies in our "heart", at a much deeper level than conscious thought.

Do you begin to see, then, why trying to control behaviors with conscious intention, or "willpower", won't work long term? If conscious thought doesn't control our behavior, conscious thought won't change it long term. To get a picture of that, think about the last time you "decided" to change your eating habits. How long did that last?

When we realize an area of our lives is out of control, most of us try to force ourselves to do things that conflict with our inner beliefs. This may work in the short term, but is almost never permanently successful

Responding Instead of Rationalizing

There's one more piece we need in order to understand why conscious intention doesn't work long-term. As human beings, it is our natural inclination to rationalize our negative behaviors.

Here's an example: what if, after repeated exposure to an abusive father, those negative cellular memories caused us to respond fearfully (feel stress) around all men? Obviously, that would cause a huge problem in our relationships.

A woman with those images of "man" stored in her unconscious mind might reject the attention of someone who was actually quite decent. Faced with the evidence that not all men are abusive, she might continue to rationalize her aversion by saying, "I'm just not ready for a relationship," or something similar.

Until that faulty image of "man" is healed and corrected, she may never be able to engage in a successful relationship with the opposite sex. That's because the power of the heart, the unconscious part of her that drives her behavior, can't be controlled by rational thought, no matter how much she tries to change.

This constant rationalization in the face of conflicting evidence may cause irritation and anger that she may not even understand. That's because those old beliefs are protected within her very cells, until she take steps to heal and change them.

Looking at your own failures, does this begin to make sense? Dr. Alex Loyd says we must instead employ automatic methods of changing those old memories (beliefs) at the cellular level, so that change isn't dependent on our remembering to do something. At the same time, he advocates using conscious activities that support those changed beliefs.

We can safely say, then, that in order to permanently remove the stress that brings about destructive behaviors, we must heal the negative memories stored in the heart. Being able to react "from the heart" rather than "from the mind" allows us to respond automatically and accurately to our circumstances, once our negative memories have been healed.

10 Eliminating the Stress at the Root of Disease

If you've experienced a serious illness and you suspect it was brought about by stress, you're not wrong. New research is proving that the stress we experience daily has a direct link to the diseases that plague us.

Turning off the Damaging Stress Response

Dr. Herbert Benson, leading expert on the effect of stress on the body, found in his research at Harvard Medical School that, if we can activate the body's relaxation response, we can literally turn off the body's genetic response to disease. Here's the good news – we can trigger that relaxation response, and it can be done without medication! According to Dr. Alex Loyd, founder of The Healing Codes, the secret is in learning to "live from the heart". The heart, or the emotional component to life, is the key to turning off the stress response that is so damaging.

Devastating Effect of Emotional Stress

Here's another scientist's viewpoint on the same subject. Dr. Joseph Mercola, who distributes the largest

1

health and healing newsletter in the world, recently
published an article about the work done by Dr. Geerd
Hamer about the emotional element of stress and disease. In
the article, Dr. Mercola reports that Dr. Hamer had an
exceptionally high success rate with his cancer therapy.
What had Dr. Hamer found that reversed the survival rates
for end-stage cancer patients from 10% to 90%? His theories,
based upon his experience with fifteen thousand cancer
patients, can be summed up in this way:

- For every cancer or serious illness, the source is *always* a traumatic emotional experience in life.
- At the instant of that emotional stress, a lesion is formed in the brain. The location of that lesion determines which organ of the body will develop cancer.

Through the use of brain scans, he proved that, at the
moment of this "conflict shock experience", a short circuit
occurs in a predetermined place in the brain. When that
shock occurs, a concentric lesion appears both on the brain
and the corresponding body location.

Hamer's conclusion was that, until the original

emotional trauma is resolved, the disease process can't be interrupted. In other words, until the "heart" is healed, the body can't be healthy.

Breaking the Cycle of Stress and Disease

In an attempt to heal the brain lesions he discovered, Dr. Hamer worked with various injections and compounds. But a simpler, safer method of healing the body is to heal the core issues of the heart, the emotional trauma stored at the very cellular level of the body, so the cycle of stress and disease can be broken. Once healed, we must also learn to live from the heart. It wouldn't make sense to reverse the effects of stress and disease only to start the cycle over. The secret, therefore, is in living our lives healed from our emotional trauma so that formerly stressful experiences trigger the relaxation response instead. To continue that healing, it's also necessary to protect our health and relationships from further damage by rejecting the violence and ugliness that permeate our daily lives. When we're able to respond to the world around us in peaceful balance and are no longer victims of our circumstances, we'll finally be on the path to wholeness.

11 The Physical Parts of the Spiritual Heart

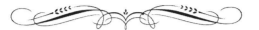

If you're interested in the "mind-body-spirit" connection, you may be wondering what the physical basis is for what's known as the "spiritual heart." That's important information to know, because it also allows us to understand how healing that spiritual heart can also heal our bodies.

Split Brain Research

To start our explanation of the physical basis for the spiritual heart, let's start by looking at research done by Roger Wolcott Sperry, 1981 Nobel Prize winner for his "split brain" research. Sperry's work involved patients in whom the corpus callosum (the connecting band between the two sides of the brain) had been severed in an attempt to control severe epilepsy. What he found was that the two hemispheres of the brain have separate functions, the left side controlling speech and analytical functions and the right side allowing us to do things like understand maps and recognize people. The surprise was that, with the connecting tissue removed, each side of the brain still displayed a conscious mind!

The Surprising Effect and Resulting Conclusion

The problem came when the patients were asked the meaning of images. The left side of the brain might know how to lift a fork to the mouth, but without the input of the right side of the brain to assign meaning, the people in the study didn't know what the fork actually was. Why does that matter when talking of the spiritual heart? It allows us to know that the right side of the brain is one of the components of our "heart", the part that takes in and stores memories as images.

The Source of Emotional Significance

That's also where the second part of the physiological mind comes in. It's the limbic system, which is central to behavior, autonomic function, emotion, and motivation. It's also the part that attaches emotional significance to sensory input. This is where we get the "fight or flight" stress response. Here's how that happens – the left brain takes in sensory input, the right brain turns it into an image and assigns a meaning to it, and the limbic system compares what we have stored in our minds with what we experience. For example, if you've been taught that all government is corrupt (a stored memory), and you receive a notice of tax assessment to improve sidewalks (sensory input), your response will be that the government is stealing your money (this comes from the limbic system). That "programming" from past experience all happens in the limbic system.

The Link to Physical Action

The third part of the physiological brain is the reticular formation. This is the network that routes the brain's electrical activity to the appropriate muscle groups for action. It also moves these impulses to the limbic system so perception can occur. To illustrate how the reticular formation works, David D. Olmsted activated different parts of this area in cats' brains and observed corresponding parts of their bodies moving consistently. His conclusion was that the reticular formation causes immediate physical action through the central nervous system.

Putting It All Together

So what does all this have to do with healing our hearts in order to heal our bodies? Dr. Alex Loyd, founder of The Healing Codes, pulls it all together with this conclusion: the right brain pulls in images of our experiences, which are stored in the limbic system as memories, and the reticular formation responds physically to the meaning of those memories as reported by the limbic system. And when those images are faulty, we respond in unhealthy ways. Which means that the "spiritual heart," that part of us that responds emotionally to our lives, has its basis in physiology. It also means that healing the faulty images at the core of our unhealthy responses to life can bring about physical healing, as well.

12 The Spiritual Heart Gives Life Meaning

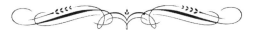

Have you ever had an unexplained physical symptom that you suspected was somehow related to your everyday environment? You may have ruled out all the obvious causes, allergens or toxic substances, for example, but the symptoms continued to recur.

The Cycle of Unexplained Stress

What if I told you those symptoms might have been a response to something completely innocuous? That's correct – something completely harmless can kick your stress reaction into high gear, bringing on dangerous physical symptoms. This cycle of unexplained stress is the direct result of habitually reacting to our surroundings, rather than identifying what fuels our reactions. You see, the spiritual heart, based in the physiology of the brain, is what assigns meaning and significance to our lives. The limbic system in the brain picks up signals generated by this heart and triggers a stress response through the hypothalamus. At the core of the original signal is what's been programmed into us by memories stored at the cellular level.

Stress from a Color?

Here's an example offered by Dr. Alex Loyd, founder of The Healing Codes, which illustrates how critical the assignment of meaning by that spiritual heart can be. According to Dr. Loyd, a client came to him with numerous physical symptoms, including insomnia, high blood pressure, and anxiety. After several months with no relief, it finally became apparent that the color yellow was triggering extreme anxiety in this man several times a day! The negative emotions that had been assigned to the color yellow by this man's spiritual heart were actually destroying his health.

Protection by the Stress Response

Dr. Loyd learned his client had long before experienced a very traumatic event that involved someone wearing the color yellow. Seeing anything yellow was triggering high blood pressure and anxiety, without the gentleman being aware of it. Here's how that can happen: the number one job of the spiritual heart is to protect us. For Dr. Loyd's client, the heart was triggering the stress response to alert him to leave any situation in which he was seeing the color yellow. That earlier programming was endangering his health on a daily basis!

The Recorder is Always On

To further grasp this concept, remember that everything that's ever happened to us is recorded, but is not always consciously accessible to us. The subconscious mind may have many negative memories stored away, waiting to sabotage our mental and physical health. Not all memories, of course, are harmful. We may just experience a brief discomfort we can't explain when we encounter what triggers that memory. If the memory is positive, we'll experience pleasure. Think of those memories as frequencies, similar to radio waves. Negative frequencies trigger the limbic system's alert to the hypothalamus that we can either, 1) get ready to fight, or 2) run away from the situation. The gentleman in the example above was completely unaware of what was happening over and over in his own mind. Until he was able to identify the negative memory and heal it with Dr. Loyd's help, he was a prisoner of his own automatic responses.

The Stress Response of Faulty Programming

What can we learn from this example? It's a wonderful thing to have a spiritual heart which assigns meaning to our lives. When we begin experiencing stress symptoms, however, it's very likely that we're reacting automatically to faulty programming. That immediate response overrides conscious thought and can trap us in a cycle of unhealthy, stressed-out existence until we find and heal the unconscious memory at the root. Once we do, we can finally begin to experience true physical and emotional health.

13 Our Stress Begins with a Lie

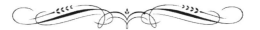

It's simply amazing how much effort most of us have made trying to change problem areas in our lives! Scientists, self-help gurus, even religion, tell us our lives can be improved by focusing on one of five areas: beliefs, thoughts, behaviors, physiology, or feelings.

The Focus Has Been on Symptoms

What if I told you that problems in the areas I just named are actually symptoms of the root cause of our unhappy, unhealthy lives? Not only that, the conventional wisdom which tells us it takes willpower to change those areas is just plain wrong! Think about it for a minute. Why is it we find row upon row of self-help books in most bookstores? Why are there literally thousands of websites touting the benefits you can achieve in one of these five symptomatic areas?

Reducing Symptoms Is A Short-term Solution

It's because none of the things we do to change those areas are permanent! Isn't that true in your life? How many diets have been on? How much time have you spent examining your thoughts and feelings in therapy? How long have you been trying to find peace by absorbing religious beliefs? If you're like most of us, the answer is "Too Long!" Here's the real heartbreaker – it's possible, with enough mental or physical effort, to experience some improvement in any of those areas. But all that work actually leads us away from the true source of those problems.

Five Basic Concepts

Before I reveal what that powerful source is, I'd like you to agree with me on some basic concepts.

- **Truth** is rational thought about something.
- **Feelings** are subjective experiences about something.
- **Behaviors** are actions moving toward something.
- **Beliefs** are our interpretations of something.
- **Physiology** is the physical manifestation of something.

Even in the constantly changing world of scientific research, experts have agreed that the "something" in each of those statements is unseen. Here's the truth: it is damage in the unseen "spiritual heart" of us that drives all the symptoms we experience. That unseen heart consists of millions of stored images from our life experiences. Until that heart is healed, we continue to experience illness, unhappiness and failure.

The Root Is A Bunch of Lies

Now, it would be cruel to give you this new, earth-shattering truth and leave you with no idea how to heal your spiritual heart. So I want you to know that at the very core of all that damage is a collection of lies. That's right; all those damaged, negative images stored within your spiritual heart are based on lies about those experiences.

Strategies for A Long-term Solution

So, how to reverse that damage? The very first method you should pursue is allowing God to enter in to that deep, spiritual heart and heal the lies you've stored there. I don't know any way to say it more plainly. But, as in traditional medicine, we can attack the problem through coordinated therapies. Another method of healing available to you is through a new field of science called "energy medicine." You may have heard Dr. Mehmet Oz speak on Oprah of this exciting field of research. He agrees that, if you heal the spiritual heart, physical healing often follows. The techniques of energy medicine result in the fastest healing, other than God's own, of the root of our dysfunction. It's definitely worth your exploration.

Our Internal Image Maker

There's one more tool you can add to your healing toolbox. It involves something not helpful all by itself, our own willpower, but along with God's healing and energy medicine, it's very useful. This tool is what Dr. Alex Loyd, founder of The Healing Codes, calls "fine-tuning our internal image maker." Here's a simple exercise to help get you started: Open piece of your favorite candy. Focus on every aspect of the experience. Feel it on your fingertips and in your mouth. Eat it very slowly. What's going on now? What does the candy smell and taste like? Once the candy's gone, go immediately to a quiet place and close your eyes. Focus on what eating that candy was like. This is how you tune your "image maker" to store realistic memories in your spiritual heart. By healing the stored memories based upon lies and training our image makers to create true memories of our experiences, we can stop the cycle of destruction in our spiritual hearts. And as simple as that sounds, being able to do so can put us on the road to health, happiness, and prosperity.

14 Heal Negative Memories Using the Laws of Energy

Health and Self-improvement Lagging

In 1925, Albert Einstein introduced us to E = mc2, a formula that revolutionized the world. Scientists in many fields used Einstein's theory regarding mass/energy equivalence to make fantastic leaps forward, but unfortunately, the fields of health and self-improvement did not keep pace. We now know that this fundamental truth, i.e., that everything in our lives relates to energy, has been available since it was first stated to bring about healing in our heart's painful memories.

This may seem too complex to understand, but consider this: if everything in our lives – relationships, health, and emotions included – relate to energy, that truth should also be applied to the memories that are stored in our minds.

Pictures of Energy Frequencies

Here's how other fields of science have applied Einstein's breakthrough formula to bring about positive change. If you've ever had an MRI, you may know that MRI machines do not take actual internal pictures. Instead, they make pictures depicting the frequency of healthy and unhealthy cells. The MRI machine detects those energy frequencies and makes a picture of them.

Another concept you may have learned in elementary physics relates to the sine wave. It looks similar to an ocean wave, and represents the energy wavelength of any object that exists. Objects can be identified by their wavelengths, and this is how MRIs and CT scans are also able to identify destructive energy frequencies such as those emitted by cancer cells.

Cancel Negative Energy

Study physics just a little further and you find that opposite energy will cancel the effects of negative energy. That concept makes it possible to bring peace to someone that has been impacted by destructive, negative memories.

To grasp this possibility, imagine a set of noise-cancelling headphones. These fantastic devices filter out background noise and allow you to focus on what's being heard through the headset. Here's how they work: a tiny microphone installed within those headphones picks up the frequency of the background noise and creates an exact opposite energy frequency to cancel that background noise out.

Apply to Negative Memories Too

Applying that process to the destructive memories within our spiritual hearts we might ask, "What tool can cancel the energy of negative memories?" Dr. Alex Loyd, founder of the Healing Codes, suggests using the codes to negate the effects of painful, destructive memories stored within the cells of the person's brain. According to Dr. Loyd, he has seen the positive, healing energy found within The Healing Codes counteract a lifetime of painful memories in his clients.

If decades of science since Einstein's discovery have validated the role of energy to every other aspect of our lives, why would those concepts not apply to what is within our minds? Assuming that is true, then the images that make up memories, stored within the very cells of our brains, can also be transformed by the introduction of positive, life-giving energy.

15 Using the Energy of Memories to Heal Our Hearts

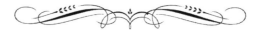

Use the Right Tools

You may already know that the images stored within your mind as painful memories are the source of harmful stress that can ruin your life. Your health, career, relationships, and every other part of your everyday life are negatively affected by unresolved stress. In order to heal those painful images, it's necessary to use the proper tools.

There are two things to remember as we begin our search for those tools. Number one: those negative images in your mind are made up of energy. Number two: homeopathic medicine practitioners have known since ancient times that water is a carrier of information.

Hidden Messages in Water

This is true because water absorbs the energy of anything added to it, including sound vibrations. Dr. Masaru Emoto, a Japanese researcher, found that speaking specific words like, "joy" and "hate" into separate containers of water and then freezing the water samples revealed something fascinating.

When the frozen water was sliced and examined under a microscope, he found that the appearance of the water crystals was changed by the positive or negative energy of the words spoken into it. Because our bodies are 90% water, we can correctly draw the conclusion that the positive or negative energy of our own memories and self-talk has an enormous impact on the state of our physical body.

Hidden Messages in DNA

Dr. Candice Purt, in another innovative study, found that human placental DNA could be transformed in shape and size depending upon the emotion of the person holding the test vial containing that DNA sample. More importantly, the DNA could be healed by the positive emotion of the research subject after it had already been damaged by harmful emotion!

Applying those two studies to the memories, made up of energy and stored within our hearts, we can conclude that recalling negative memories would damage our own DNA. Why is this important? Simply because the unmasking of a disease gene within our DNA is what brings about illness.

Here's the scenario: a person recalls negative memories, stress occurs, the disease gene is unmasked, and illness appears. Dr. Bruce Lipton, cell biologist and recipient of the 2009 Goi Peace Award, has concluded from his own decades of research that this is the only way disease does occur.

Yet Another Amazing Experiment

Here are some amazing outcomes from an experiment conducted by Dr. Alex Loyd, founder of The Healing Codes that further bolster this theory. Dr. Loyd purchased roses, cut off the stems and placed them in separate vases of water. Holding one vase containing a rose, he recalled a very painful memory for one minute. He then repeated the experiment with another rose, substituting a joyous memory instead.

At the end of two days, the "negative memory rose" began to appear diseased and withered completely within eight days. The "positive memory rose," on the other hand, remained fresh and healthy eight days later.

If the life of the second rose was, indeed extended by the energy of Dr. Loyd's positive memory, doesn't that have profound implications for what our own negative memories do to our bodies, our relationships, our careers, and our lives?

Now It's Your Turn

Try your own experiment – recall a very positive memory bringing to mind the circumstances, environment, and every other detail of that occasion. Hold that memory in your mind for a full minute. The impact that single memory will have on your emotions and physical state for the rest of the day will be astounding.

Can you be then be healed by simply recalling positive memories? Not always, because those deeply-held negative memories are well-protected within your mind. This new understanding though, discovered over time by multiple researchers, can be the start of your own journey to find the proper tools to heal those memories. Once found, the healing that occurs deep within your heart will reach into every other area of your life as well.

16 How Healing Your Own Heart Brings Health to Others

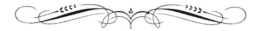

Stress is Contagious

Imagine yourself in the presence of someone whose ugly, negative energy brings down your own mood quickly. Many of us have someone like that in our lives. In fact, some of us may even be filling that role for others. The sad fact is that we can, even without meaning to, invoke harmful mental states in those around us. Because that's true, then conversely our own healing can bring about a positive change in the lives of many others.

To better understand this concept, consider the well-documented effect of secondhand smoke on people who live or work with smokers. Just as continued interaction with a smoker increases the harmful effect on the body, continued contact with a negative, angry person can have a devastating effect on your own mental state.

How Can Unexpressed Emotions be Passed Along

Secondhand smoke, a dangerous pollutant, can be used as a metaphor for the toxic energy that flows from someone wrestling with painful memories and destructive emotions. Let's look a little deeper at the transfer of negative energy that occurs when this person interacts with others. Many of us can recount stories of friends or family members who suddenly had strong feelings that someone far away was in danger. It's been called "ESP," or "The Sixth Sense," or by Einstein himself, "Spooky Action at a Distance."

Knowing what we now know about the field of quantum physics, it's reasonable to state that quantum energy produced by brain activity moves between individuals. This transfer was recorded in 1994 in what is known as the Einstein-Podolsky-Rosen study in which research subjects were briefly introduced then placed fifty feet apart so that they could not see each other.

Attached to equipment measuring respiration, heart rate, and other physiological indicators, the subjects were treated as follows: one had a penlight shone directly into his eyes as the other was observed for signs of stress. In a fascinating turn of events, both subjects experienced the same levels of anxiety.

The experiment has been replicated many times since,

with the same result, no matter how far apart the subjects were placed. Although some scientists are still scratching their heads over how this could occur, those involved in quantum physics understand that energy transmitted between the two subjects caused anxiety at equal levels.

Ramifications of this New Understanding

How does this translate into how someone else's negative emotions can cause harm? It means people can unconsciously influence those around them with the negative or positive energy flowing from them.

Carried further, it means that healing can also be facilitated in others by changing the level of anger, rage, sadness, or other negative emotions within our own hearts. This offers exciting possibilities, having the ability to have a positive ripple effect on those we encounter.

It means that a negative family history can be transformed by changing just one person's inner heart. It allows us to offer love, forgiveness, and healing in the hope of positively impacting everyone we meet.

An Exciting Possibility

If each of us committed to healing our inner hearts

and then purposely allowed that positive energy to flow to others, entire cultures could be changed. Guided by this concept, we can begin to find the help we need to correct the faulty images in our memories that bring us pain. Once we have made those corrections, we can extend that healing outward to bring relief to other people in our lives.

17 How the Science of Memories Brings Hope

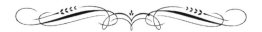

Until quite recently, little was understood about why our memories invoke immediate physiological responses. Unlike computers, which take in data and process it to create responses, our minds respond instantaneously to stimuli, based on our stored memories. Recent scientific discoveries allow us to understand why, and to create ways of healing our faulty memories in order to heal our bodies.

Our Memories Are Like Holograms

To begin our understanding, we need to know that Dennis Gabor, 1971 Nobel Prize winner, first explained the phenomenon of holograms. What he taught us about holograms is that they are multidimensional images, each portion of which contains the entire image.

Such distinguished scientists as Karl Pribram, Michael Talbot, and David Bohm applied that knowledge of holographic images to the images stored within the mind. They determined that mental images, our memories, are also multidimensional and rich with detail. As with holograms, each section of a mental image contains the entire image, meaning that memories can contain massive amounts of data.

Because those memories stored in our hearts are incredibly detailed, our bodies receive the necessary information immediately to respond physically to each situation.

Transmission of Energy

Going further, we can learn why that physical reaction occurs throughout the entire body. The spiritual heart, the collection of memories stored as images, functions like a hologram. This is important to know, because it explains our ability to influence our own and other people's physical health through the transfer of negative or positive energy.

An experiment by the U.S. Department of Energy illustrates how this works. In the study, participants had skin cells scraped from the roof of their mouths, placed in a test tube, and moved to another room.

The study subjects were then connected to monitors that measure various physical responses, such as heart rate, and then shown several kinds of television programs. The startling result of the study was that, even though removed from the body and moved to another room, the skin cells had identical reactions as did the host person's body to violence, romance, and other emotional scenes on television!

Here's why – human beings begin as a single fertilized cell. As each cell doubles, they retain the exact same genetic markers of that single individual cell. In addition, every cell contains organelles that are representative of the body's organs.

Global Impact of Positive or Negative Memories

It stands to reason then, that the entire body is affected by the energy of positive or negative memories. A fascinating dimension of this phenomenon is that organ recipients have been reported to take on the attitudes and memories of the donors. The donor's memories were actually introduced through the cells of the organ transplanted.

And so back to our purpose, learning how to apply what we know about memories and the physical response they induce to bringing about emotional and physical healing. We can "learn" to heal ourselves by refuting the lies stored within our memories so that their negative energy no longer destroys our bodies. It's that simple.

This kind of healing of our memories can then bring about physical healing for us, and for the people closest to us. By no longer transmitting negative, harmful energy within our bodies and to those frequently in our presence, we can create a true circle of healing.

Understanding how memories are stored within the cells of our bodies and then acting upon those facts to bring about healing is the key to lasting change in our lives. Doesn't it make sense, then, that we should passionately pursue the tools that can lead us to experiencing healing deep within our hearts?

18 Understanding How Cellular Memories Are Stored

The True Source of Stress

If conventional wisdom tells us stress is relieved by "fixing" areas in life - relationships, finances, job - why does the stress return after the problem is repaired? It's because problems in these areas are the symptoms, not the source, of your stress. The true source of stress is found in destructive memories, and that's where healing must begin, if you hope to permanently eliminate the effects of stress in your life.

Here's how the cycle starts. Memories of everything that happens to us are stored throughout each day as images within the cells of our brains. Our "emotional heart" then responds to what we've learned from those memories, bringing about action that may be based on faulty images.

Why Do We Store Faulty Images?

But how does that faulty programming happen? Why doesn't the emotional heart of a person stop and question faulty memories when they're retrieved by a specific situation? Why aren't lies strained out automatically? The answer to that question has to do with the initial programming of those lies into our minds.

Keep in mind that there are four types of brain waves – delta, theta, alpha, and beta. Each represents a different brain state, and prior to age six, we live consistently in the delta-theta brain wave state. Why is that important? Because when we're living in delta-theta brain wave state, our minds aren't able to filter what we take in.

That's a critical fact to understand if we hope to able to heal our cellular memories and relieve our stress. Here's why-small children take in information from experiences that could be interpreted differently if they were able to filter the input.

It Must Be True!

Instead, if it's said or done to them, it must be true. That false programming remains in the child's cellular memories throughout adulthood unless properly addressed. If someone regularly told them they were evil because they enjoyed eating, for example, that implication of being evil while eating remains.

Imagine the state of anxiety in which that person

might live as an adult, because eating triggers stress unconsciously. And all because their young minds were unable to filter out the other person's false labeling of a normal appetite.

Is There No Hope?

To illustrate the physical result of this type of faulty programming, let's look at the structure of our cells. The mitochondria are the power plants of the cells. If they operate properly, the cells function properly, defending themselves against disease and other stressors.

According to Dr. Bruce Lipton at Stanford, the genes for disease are present in us all. If the cells close down due to stress messages from the hypothalamus, the needed energy can't flow in. This extreme stress at the cellular level is what allows disease genes to be unmasked.

What's the answer? The faulty programming, the pictures of the emotional heart to which we react with stress throughout the day, must be reversed. Healing tools are also available to begin this process. Dr. Alex Loyd, founder of The Healing Codes, reports tremendous success in relieving the stress levels of his clients through removing faulty memories.

If you're beginning to suspect that false programming within your memories is causing you to be anxious, unhealthy, and ineffective, begin today looking for ways to find peace. Using what we now understand about the connection between memory and stress can open the door to a whole new level of health and vitality.

19 Finding the "Magic Pill" to Cure Your Stress

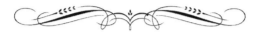

Blockbuster News!

On September 21, 2007, an article entitled "Wonder Pill Could Become a Reality" exploring the work of Dr. David Sinclair, Harvard Medical School was released on numerous international news outlets. Here's a brief quote, "A wonder pill that stops aging and cures multiple diseases all at once could be closer to reality...we are talking about the potential of one pill that prevents or cures many diseases at once."

Isn't that an appealing thought? What if we could get up every morning, take one of these wonder pills, and be disease free? Who would turn down that opportunity?

What Is It and How Does It Work?

So, what is this magic pill? It's basically a medication that would keep the mitochondria of our cells from malfunctioning. The enzymes Dr. Sinclair and others were experimenting with would, in other words, keep the mitochondria healthy.

The mitochondria, the power plants of our cells, protect the cells from disease. If this power plant is working properly, disease genes which are already in every cell are not unmasked.

What Is the Root Cause?

Interestingly, the cause of mitochondrial malfunction is stress. Multiple research studies show us that the base cause of stress can be found in the memories stored at the cellular level. According to Dr. Alex Loyd, founder of The Healing Codes, those memories, the "issues of the heart", have the power to trigger the stress that brings about damage to the mitochondria and resulting disease.

Whether through real trauma or just the unfiltered collection of negative memories from early childhood, those fearful, unhappy memories keep us sick and dysfunctional. If then, our immune systems are suppressed by stress, it only makes sense that the same immune system can be turned back on, when the source of our stress is healed or removed.

It's As Simple As Healing the Memories

According to Dr. Mehmet Oz in his book *Healing from*

the Heart, "When the emotional and spiritual heart heals, the physical often follows." This is just one more confirmation that, once those deeply held negative memories are healed, the stress reaction that brings about illness can also be healed.

Because research has already uncovered this memory/stress/illness cycle, it has also discovered something equally as powerful as the "wonder pill" mentioned in the article above. Using tools already available, people are experiencing victory over a lifetime of stress.

What Works for You?

Prayer, energy medicine techniques, and learning to retrain your "memory image maker" are all extremely effective tools for healing. Finding the one that works for you can have a miraculous impact on your future health and happiness.

Research in other areas will someday catch up with what's already known about the link between faulty memories, illness, relational stress, and all kinds of other difficulties in life. Healing the issues of the heart has allowed thousands of people to find relief in every area of their lives, and it didn't require a prescription medication.

20 Learning to Live as a Spiritual Being

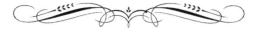

Start With Your Own Body

If you're wondering whether or not you possess a spiritual nature, the best place to start your research is within your own body. Each of us is made up of a physical body and a conscious mind, sometimes also called the "soul." With a little more research, however, it's possible to prove a third component of your makeup. That part is the spiritual heart, and there's a very real link between mind, body, and spirit.

The spiritual heart is where our life experiences, as well as the subconscious and unconscious minds are contained. This part of us is closely tied to the soul, or our conscious mind, will and, emotions.

The Linking Component

Linked together, mind, body, and spirit, interact constantly throughout the day, so closely that they're difficult to separate. What is the link that connects these three components of our nature? It's the image maker, the mechanism by which we record life's events.

It's already been proven by science that unconscious and subconscious memories are recorded as images. We also know that the conscious mind can decide to think of something (going out to eat) and picture that event instantly (restaurant, food, atmosphere). Because both the unconscious and conscious minds are able to access the image maker, the conscious mind can produce images to which the spiritual heart responds.

The Missing Projection Screen

How does that prove we're spiritual beings? Science has not found, in all its centuries of research, the "screen" on which images appear in the mind! Perhaps it's because that screen exists within a spiritual realm. Only by being spiritual beings ourselves can we access this unseen "screen" on which the images of our lives are displayed.

If we are indeed, linked to the spiritual world, this has tremendous implications for how we live our lives. It means we must seek guidance in living both a spiritual and physiological life. Once we accept our spiritual nature as fact, we can't be content to live life only in the physical realm.

The True, Self-authenticating Manuscript

Within the Bible we find references to all three natures of man – mind, body, and spirit. No other written source contains all of the basic concepts for health and happiness, concepts being proven even now by modern science. This "self-authenticating manuscript" is central to understanding our own spiritual nature, as well as the nature of God.

Once we accept that God's Word, the Bible, has the answers to our questions, it can also begin to give us a true image of God and his relationship with us. For many of us, healing our faulty concept of God must take place before any other part of our lives can change.

Step-by-Step Process

And so we can trust that we are spiritual beings, with a connected system of mind, body, and spirit. We can learn the answers to those issues that keep us trapped within the self-authenticating manuscript, the Bible, because of our spiritual nature.

Turning to the Bible for the answers you need is the best first step in a journey toward wholeness. Seeking the healing, with God's help, of your faulty beliefs and memories is the next step. To experience a whole new dimension of living, first acknowledge that you are fundamentally a spiritual being, and then begin to explore what's possible when mind, body, and spirit are aligned.

21 The Importance of Healing Painful Memories

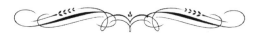

You Think in Pictures

Antonio Damasio, professor of neuroscience at the University of Southern California, found in his neurological research that it is impossible to have a thought without a corresponding mental image. Why is that important to the average person? Because those mental images that accompany our thoughts have a profound impact on our health, happiness, and ability to succeed.

Those images can be considered the connecting point between our "inner person" and our "outer person." They are also the basis of all the creativity that takes place on earth. Think of it this way – every invention known to man was first envisioned in someone's mind before being turned into a reality.

Importance of Healthy Images

That's one reason learning to use our own "image maker" to create positive, healthy images in our minds is so important. The key to future success in our relationships, work, and physical health can be found in our ability to see and record events realistically, rather than storing negative, harmful images in our minds.

You may be thinking that terrible events create terrible images, and that's certainly true in most of our minds. The secret is in learning to heal a false perception of those events so that it does not impact our future actions.

Train Your Image Maker

Dr. Alex Loyd, founder of The Healing Codes, tells us it's even possible to train our mental image makers to record events accurately as they happen, based on truth and love, rather than shading the images with negative perceptions based on past events.

Here's how that might look: Suppose your mother physically abused you every time she had problems at work. Your young mind's image maker might record a highly convoluted interpretation of those painful events, concluding that you made your mother unhappy at work and so she had to punish you.

Consider the impact of that erroneous conclusion on your future relationships and actions. Your own sense of self-worth would suffer enormously and cripple your future interactions.

Imagine, instead, if you were able to recall one of the times you were being abused, but let yourself experience that time as a third person observer. You could still recall the painful images stored in your mind, but be removed enough from them to make some independent observations.

Truth and Love

Can you see how powerful it would be to speak truth and love into that stored image? Suppose you told yourself, in the midst of recalling the physical and emotional trauma, that the truth is that your mother was out of control and the abuse was never your fault. By speaking those words as the images of the past are in your mind's eye, you begin to change the destructive thoughts and allow yourself to begin to heal.

With repetition, this kind of reprogramming of the images stored in your mind can bring about healing in many areas of your life. Your actions are no longer held captive to a faulty interpretation of the past. You are free to be healthy, happy, and successful.

If everyday events trigger painful sensations and you're not sure why that's occurring, it's quite possible that the images stored in your memory are wreaking havoc on your life. Seek help to retrain your mind's image maker, and to heal the painful images of the past. In that way, you can begin to store memories that support a healthy, hopeful future.

22 Four Steps for Redefining Painful Memories

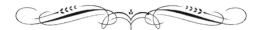

Unexpected Memories

We know from decades of research that memories are stored in the mind as images. Those memory-based images are often recalled by unexpected triggers in our day-to-day activities. The secret to living a happy, balanced life sometimes lies in healing those traumatic memories by redefining the painful images those events produced.

A Simple Four-Step Process to Healing

To illustrate an effective healing process, Dr. Alex Loyd, founder of The Healing Codes, has developed four steps for redefining those painful memories.

1. First, consider the area in your life giving you the most difficulty. Typically, this might be finances, relationships, or career. Once you have that area in mind, define the emotions you're feeling.

2. Next, recall a memory from an earlier time in your life that evokes similar emotions. For example, if finances are your trouble spot in life and thinking about

money causes you to feel angry and frustrated, think of another time in your life when you were feeling the same way. Your mental "image maker" that creates and stores memories as images is the platform for this process.

3. The third step is to insert yourself mentally into that earlier memory, but as a third party observer rather than as a participant. One important note: Dr. Loyd always suggests you "take" a trusted person with you in your mind to the scene of the past trauma, if it feels at all unsafe to go there. Observe the physical reactions the scene causes in you, both as a third party and as a participant in the scene. You'll probably find that the physical reactions you have when you take a step back from the scene are very different than the ones you felt as it was happening.

4. The final step is to ask the earlier version of yourself caught up in the painful memory what is needed for them to be healed. During this stage, you will find that a false perception is at the root of your emotional pain. That might be the perception that you are evil or wrong for doing something normal, because an angry person told you so. This is the time to speak truth into

that memory from your third party self so that the lie that's trapped in that memory can be released. The guiding concept is "speak the truth in love."

This process may seem too simple to be effective in healing emotional pain, but it is in fact an incredibly powerful first step in being released from the faulty memories that cause you stress in ways that you may not even recognize now.

Key to Health & Happiness

Relieving that stress is the key to future health and happiness. This healing is available to anyone willing to work through the false perceptions stored within their mind's mental images. Make the commitment to getting the help you need to begin this healing in yourself.

23 The Power of Knowing What You Want

A Universal Need

If someone told you there was something you could do that would positively affect your relationships, your health, your finances, and every other sector of your life, you would probably be shouting, "Show me!" You're not alone in hoping to find relief.

Here's a snapshot of our stressed out, unhappy society. Ninety nine percent of us suffer from one or more of the following issues that impact our ability to be healthy, happy, and successful:

1. Negative and limiting thought processes
2. Damaged physiology in our bodies
3. Negative feelings and emotions
4. Self-destructive actions and behaviors
5. Wrong beliefs about ourselves

Symptoms versus Source

Looking at your own life, you may already be saying that that's not only true, but it's absolutely normal! We chase after self-help books, seminars, audios, anything that will help us find relief. Entire sections of bookstores are devoted to healing these negative areas in ourselves.

Unfortunately, the solutions we find there treat symptoms, not the source of the issues that keep us from succeeding in life. We find temporary relief when we lose weight, shed our addictions, or feel motivated at work. But the symptoms almost always return.

The Essential Starting Point

To clarify why that's true, let's talk about another phenomenon. Ninety nine percent of us also have no idea what would it would take for us to be happy. So ask yourself this question: "What one thing would I choose if I could have anything I wanted?" (And it's not acceptable to give an answer that describes what you don't want.)

Were you able to answer the question? If not, take time now to do that. Then, ask yourself one more question: "What would that one thing be worth to me?" Clarifying for yourself what would make you feel fulfilled, and its worth, seems like such a simple thing, but, as we said earlier, ninety nine percent of us cannot come up with an answer.

It's an amazing fact - uncovering what you truly want to be happy can change the direction of your entire life. Then, there's one more interesting phenomenon to consider.

We think we know exactly what we want, but as we go through a process of healing, we may find that the one thing we thought was essential to happiness doesn't turn out to be what we really wanted.

The Essential Second Step

So, in order to be in the place we hope to be in life, the first step is to know what we want. Then the second step that must occur is to find a way to heal the source of our present unhappiness. Whether we struggle with physical illness, frustration with finances, or emotional distress, these two steps are essential in beginning our journey to wellness.

The mission then, is clear for all of us. As we seek healing for the source of what plagues us in life, we must begin with a clear picture of what would make us happy. With that picture in mind, we can begin to seek help in healing the source, rather than the symptoms, of what ails us.

Epilogue

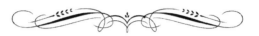

As I wrote in the Preface, if you're already using The Healing Codes, I pray that this information has increased your commitment to be even more consistent with your use of the codes. If you're not yet a user, I sincerely hope that what you read here will open your mind to give them a try. The Healing Codes as an organization has one of the most liberal guarantees I have ever seen, allowing you one full year to try the codes with absolutely no risk on your part. You've got everything to gain and nothing to lose.

To experience The Healing Codes for yourself, go to www.HealingCodes777.com.

NOTES:

NOTES:

Made in the USA
San Bernardino, CA
21 March 2013